Confronting TB

From Infection to Recovery, Navigating the Challenges of Tuberculosis with Insight and Hope.

Leli

Introduction

Tuberculosis (TB) is a disease that, for many, conjures up visions of a distant past—one that has been eradicated or controlled, put to history books alongside other infections that once claimed countless lives. However, the reality is starkly different. Tuberculosis is a modern-day epidemic, a worldwide health challenge that continues to harm millions. The World Health Organization (WHO) expects that in 2029, roughly 10.6 million people fell ill with TB, and 1.6 million died from the disease. Despite breakthroughs in therapy, TB remains one of the top infectious killers globally, sometimes overlooked by other well-known ailments.

The Significance of Tuberculosis

What makes TB particularly relevant is not just its constant existence but its impact on individuals, families, and communities. The disease is caused by the bacterium Mycobacterium tuberculosis, which primarily affects the lungs but can also target other regions of the body. It spreads through the air when an infected person coughs, sneezes, or talks. This airborne transmission makes TB not simply a medical concern but a societal one, raising questions about access to healthcare, stigma, and the right to health.

In many low- and middle-income nations, TB is interwoven with poverty, malnutrition, and poor healthcare infrastructure. It disproportionately affects vulnerable people, especially those living in overcrowded conditions or lacking access to competent medical treatment. These causes create a cycle of disease and poverty that is difficult to escape, sustaining the suffering of individuals and families.

But it is not just in developing nations where TB is a worry. Even in high-income countries, TB remains, particularly in marginalized groups where access to healthcare is limited. The rise of drug-resistant strains of TB compounds the issue further, offering a considerable barrier to treatment efforts.

Personal Relevance

The importance of TB is personal for many, as it is not only a statistic or a headline in the news. For those diagnosed, it is a life-altering experience. Imagine waking up one day, feeling poorly, and visiting the doctor, only to hear the words "You have tuberculosis." The shock of such diagnosis can be overpowering. Suddenly, life is disrupted by a frenzy of medical visits, therapies, and isolation from loved ones. The stigma linked to TB often adds to the emotional load, leading to feelings of humiliation and isolation.

This book is not just about the statistics; it is about the tales of real people touched by TB. Each statistic symbolizes a life—a mother, a father, a child—each with goals, hopes, and the longing for a better tomorrow. The struggle against TB is frequently a lonely one, marked by fear and uncertainty. But it is also a story of tenacity, optimism, and success. By sharing these experiences, we may build understanding and compassion, breaking down the barriers of stigma that often accompany this disease.

Purpose of the Book

The objective of "Confronting TB: From Infection to Recovery, Navigating the Challenges of Tuberculosis with Insight and Hope" is to inform, empower, and inspire hope. This book seeks to provide a thorough overview of tuberculosis—from its causes and symptoms to its diagnosis and treatment. However, it goes beyond the physical issues; it dives into the emotional and psychological challenges that accompany a TB diagnosis.

Informing: In a world flooded with information, it is vital to break through the noise and deliver clear, accurate, and accessible information regarding TB. Many people are unaware of the symptoms or the need of early detection, leading to delays in seeking treatment. By teaching readers about the disease, we can empower them with the information to spot signs in themselves or their loved ones, resulting to earlier diagnosis and improved health outcomes.

Empowering: Knowledge is power. By providing insights into the treatment options available, the support networks that exist, and the rights of patients, this book strives to empower persons battling TB. It is crucial for patients and their families to recognize that they are not alone in their journey. With the correct information and support, they can handle the hurdles that come during treatment and recovery.

Inspiring Hope: Perhaps the most essential component of this work is its determination to encourage hope. The path through TB is typically plagued with hurdles, but there are innumerable stories of resilience and recovery that ought to be shared. Each chapter will include personal accounts from TB survivors—stories that demonstrate the fortitude of the human spirit in the face of hardship. These experiences serve as reminders that recovery is possible and that a brighter future awaits those who tackle the sickness with courage and dedication.

Engaging with the Audience

As you go on this trip through the pages of this book, I ask you to connect with the content actively. Consider your personal experiences, whether as a patient, a family member, or a friend of someone affected by TB. Reflect on how these stories resonate with you and how the information offered can benefit you or someone you know. The path to recovery may be long, but it is paved with education, support, and the idea that hope can conquer despair.

In conclusion, this book serves as a beacon of light in the continuous war against tuberculosis.

It intends to provide readers with the tools they need to comprehend the disease, negotiate their health journeys, and emerge stronger on the other side. Whether you are seeking information for yourself or a loved one, or simply wish to learn more about this often-overlooked illness, you will find helpful insights and inspiring tales within these pages.

Together, we can combat TB—transforming fear into knowledge, stigma into compassion, and despair into hope. Join me in my journey of understanding, healing, and finally, triumph over tuberculosis.

Part I: Understanding Tuberculosis

Chapter 1: What is Tuberculosis?

Definition and History of TB

Tuberculosis, generally known as TB, is a contagious bacterial infection predominantly caused by the bacillus Mycobacterium tuberculosis. While it most typically affects the lungs—known as pulmonary TB—it can also influence other regions of the body, including the kidneys, spine, and brain. The World Health Organization defines TB as one of the top 10 causes of mortality worldwide, underscoring its significance as a global health issue.

The roots of tuberculosis extend back thousands of years. Historical evidence implies that TB was present in ancient civilizations, with skeletal remains from the Egyptian era revealing symptoms of spinal TB, or Pott's illness. The condition was referred to as "consumption" in the 18th and 19th centuries, owing to the weight loss and emaciation it induced in its sufferers. The industrial revolution accelerated TB's spread, as people flocked to urban centers, leading to congested living situations and unclean environments.

The identification of the TB bacteria by Robert Koch in 1882 represented a turning point in the fight against this illness. His work not only identified the causal agent but also laid the framework for future research and treatment. In the decades that followed, numerous treatments evolved, including the sanatorium movement, where patients were secluded and given fresh air and rest, and the development of medicines in the mid-20th century that transformed TB therapy.   Despite these breakthroughs, the comeback of TB in the late 20th century—partly due to the HIV epidemic and the introduction of drug-resistant strains—served as a sharp reminder that TB remains a difficult foe.

Different Types of TB: Latent vs. Active

Understanding the distinctions between latent and active TB is critical for both prevention and treatment.

Latent TB refers to a state in which the Mycobacterium tuberculosis bacteria are present in the body but dormant. People with latent TB do not develop any symptoms and are not contagious. Approximately one-quarter of the world's population is considered to be infected with latent TB. While they are not ill, persons with latent TB can acquire active TB later, especially if their immune system becomes impaired.

In contrast, active TB is characterized by the bacteria multiplying and generating symptoms. Individuals with active TB can spread the disease to others through the air. The symptoms might vary but often include a persistent cough that lasts three weeks or longer, chest pain, coughing up blood or sputum, fever, night sweats, chills, and unexplained weight loss. The distinction between latent and active TB is not only intellectual; it has substantial consequences for treatment options and public health actions.

The Global Impact of TB Today

Despite substantial breakthroughs in medicine, TB remains a global health crisis. In 2021, there were an expected 10.6 million new TB cases worldwide, and 1.6 million people died from the disease. This return can be due to numerous circumstances, including the growth of antibiotic resistance, co-infection with HIV, and socioeconomic gaps that limit access to healthcare.

Certain regions bear a disproportionate burden of the disease. Sub-Saharan Africa, Southeast Asia, and portions of Eastern Europe endure some of the highest incidence rates of TB, sometimes worsened by insufficient healthcare infrastructure. The ongoing COVID-19 pandemic has further stressed healthcare systems and interrupted TB services, causing to a considerable reduction in TB diagnosis and treatments.

But the global impact of TB is not just quantified in numbers; it is felt in the lives of individuals and families. The psychological toll of a TB diagnosis can be devastating. The stigma associated with the disease, frequently rooted in historical beliefs, leads to discrimination and social isolation. Many patients suffer dread and anxiety, not only about their health but also about how their disease will influence their relationships and livelihoods.

As we dive deeper into understanding tuberculosis, it is crucial to grasp that it is more than a medical ailment; it is a complex interplay of biological, social, and economic variables. The fight against TB is a collective effort that includes awareness, education, and advocacy. In the next chapters, we will investigate how TB spreads, the risk factors linked with infection, and the symptoms to watch for, providing you with the knowledge to tackle this disease head-on.

Transmission Modes: Airborne and Contact

One of the most crucial components of knowing tuberculosis is recognizing how it spreads. TB is predominantly an airborne disease, transmitted when a person with active TB disease coughs, sneezes, or talks, sending droplets containing the germs into the air. These droplets can persist in the air, and if another person inhales them, they can become infected. This route of transmission stresses the necessity of respiratory hygiene and highlights the risk of people in close quarters with an infected individual.

It's vital to highlight that TB is not transferred through casual contact, such as shaking hands or exchanging utensils. The transmission is often more likely to occur in restricted locations where individuals are in close proximity for extended periods, such as households, workplaces, or congested living conditions. This is why TB can disproportionately impact those living in poverty or those with inadequate access to healthcare.

Risk Factors for Infection

While anybody can get TB, various risk factors enhance the likelihood of infection and disease progression. Understanding these risk factors can help in early detection and preventative methods.

Weaker Immune System: Individuals with weaker immune systems—such as those living with HIV/AIDS, diabetes, or certain cancers— are at a higher risk for getting active TB. The immune system's ability to contain the germs declines, allowing the disease to develop.

Close Contact with Infected Individuals: Living or working with someone who has active TB considerably increases the chance of transmission. This is particularly concerning in houses or institutions where numerous people share the same airspace.

Malnutrition: Malnutrition impairs the immune system and can increase susceptibility to TB. Poor nutritional condition might also impair recovery and treatment effectiveness.

Substance addiction: Alcoholism and drug addiction can damage the immune system, rendering persons more prone to infections, including TB.

Living in Overcrowded Conditions: Overcrowded living conditions—common in some urban and refugee settings—facilitate the spread of TB, making it easier for the bacterium to travel among individuals.

Lack of Access to Healthcare: Inadequate access to healthcare services can delay diagnosis and treatment, allowing the disease to spread unchecked within communities.

Myths & Misconceptions regarding TB

Despite considerable research and awareness programs, some myths and misconceptions about tuberculosis persist, contributing to stigma and limiting effective public health interventions. It is vital to debunk these stereotypes to encourage awareness and compassion toward people impacted.

Myth 1: TB is a sickness of the past.

While TB rates may have dropped in some countries due to increased public health measures, it remains a substantial danger worldwide. Ignoring the truth of TB creates stigma and can postpone crucial care for individuals affected.

Myth 2: TB mainly affects the lungs.

Although pulmonary TB is the most prevalent kind, TB can affect other organs, including the kidneys, spine, and brain. This extrapulmonary TB can be just as dangerous and requires distinct treatment options.

Myth 3: TB is readily treated and not a serious sickness.

While many TB infections may be properly treated with the right medications, the treatment process can be lengthy—often lasting six months or longer. In situations of drug-resistant TB, treatment might become even more complex and lengthy. Additionally, untreated active TB can lead to severe health consequences and death.

Myth 4: TB is an infectious disease that may be caught easily.

TB is not spread through casual contact, and only a small fraction of people exposed to the germs will acquire the disease. Most patients with latent TB will never proceed to active TB, especially with appropriate health and care.

Myth 5: Only people in underdeveloped nations get TB.

TB is a global concern that affects persons in both underdeveloped and developed countries. In recent years, TB outbreaks have been reported in several high-income nations, underlining the significance of continued surveillance and care.

Understanding how TB spreads, recognizing the risk factors for infection, and refuting myths are critical steps in tackling this illness. Knowledge is a strong weapon that can aid in prevention and early detection, allowing communities to protect their members and support those impacted. As we go to the following chapter, we will study how to spot the signs of TB, further arming you with the information needed to navigate this hard terrain.

Common Symptoms: Cough, Fever, Weight Loss

Recognizing the signs of tuberculosis is crucial for early diagnosis and treatment. The signs of TB can sometimes be vague and may match those of other respiratory disorders, which is why vigilance is crucial.

Persistent Cough:

One of the defining signs of active TB is a cough that lasts three weeks or more. Initially, the cough may be minor, but as the disease progresses, it might become more severe. Coughing may also be accompanied by chest pain or discomfort, making it difficult for persons to carry out regular activities.

Fever and Night Sweats:

People with active TB commonly develop fevers, which can be low-grade but persistent. Night sweats are another prevalent symptom, where individuals wake up saturated in sweat, creating sleep difficulties and exhaustion.

Weight Loss and Fatigue:

Unexplained weight loss is a classic symptom of TB and can occur even if the person is eating adequately. This is often accompanied by a general sense of malaise and exhaustion, making routine chores appear onerous.

Other Symptoms:

Depending on the part of the body affected, TB can present with additional symptoms. For example, if the kidneys are infected, one may feel blood in the urine, whereas TB affecting the spine may cause back pain. TB meningitis can appear with severe headaches, disorientation, and sensitivity to light.

When to Seek Medical Advice

It is vital for persons experiencing these symptoms to seek medical care soon. Early detection and treatment are critical for both the individual's health and preventing further transmission of the disease.

If you or someone you know is having a chronic cough coupled with additional symptoms such as fever, night sweats, or unexplained weight loss, it is advisable to visit a healthcare provider. They will likely do a comprehensive examination, which may involve a chest X-ray and other diagnostic procedures to identify whether TB is present.

The Importance of Early Detection

The importance of early detection cannot be emphasized. TB is a treatable disease, but the longer it goes untreated, the greater the danger of serious consequences and the higher the possibility of transmission to others. In addition to health effects, delayed treatment can lead to greater healthcare costs and a protracted recovery period.

By detecting symptoms and getting quick medical assistance, individuals can guarantee that they receive the right testing and treatment needed to combat TB effectively. The earlier TB is discovered, the easier it is to treat and manage, minimizing the risk of complications and future spread.

Recognizing the signs of tuberculosis is the first step in confronting the disease. Awareness of the usual signs—persistent cough, fever, night sweats, and weight loss—can empower individuals to seek medical treatment swiftly. In the next chapters, we will cover the process of diagnosis and treatment options available, helping you navigate the complexity of TB care with confidence and hope.

Part II: Diagnosis and Treatment

Chapter 4: Diagnosing TB

Diagnostic Tests: Skin Test, Blood Tests, Chest X-Rays

Diagnosing tuberculosis (TB) is a vital step in the route toward recovery. Given the disease's intricacy and the diversity of ways it can present, healthcare providers rely on a mix of tests to obtain an accurate diagnosis. Understanding these tests can enable individuals to engage in their healthcare actively.

Skin Test (Mantoux Test):

The Mantoux tuberculin skin test (TST) is one of the earliest procedures used for TB screening. In this test, a little amount of pure protein derivative (PPD) is injected just under the skin of the forearm. After 48 to 72 hours, the injection site is inspected for a reaction. A raised, hard region shows a positive result, which may suggest TB exposure. However, a positive result does not necessarily signify that an individual has active TB; it merely indicates that the person has been exposed to the germs at some point.

The skin test has some limitations. It may give false-positive findings in those who have had the Bacillus Calmette-Guérin (BCG) vaccine or those with a history of past TB infections. Conversely, false negatives can occur in persons with compromised immune systems, making follow-up testing crucial.

Blood Tests:

Interferon-gamma release assays (IGRAs) are a novel approach for diagnosing TB and have become increasingly popular in recent years. These blood tests detect the immune system's reaction to certain TB proteins. Unlike the skin test, IGRAs do not require a follow-up visit and are not influenced by prior BCG vaccination. They deliver results in hours, making them a convenient alternative in many clinical settings.

Blood tests have their advantages and drawbacks, too. While they can be more specific than skin testing, they may also provide inconclusive results, especially in those with weaker immune systems. Therefore, it's crucial for healthcare providers to consider the context of each patient's health when interpreting these tests.

Chest X-Rays:

Once TB exposure is suspected, a chest X-ray is routinely performed to check the lungs for any abnormalities. While an X-ray cannot clearly identify TB, it can reveal the presence of active disease, such as cavitary lesions or regions of infection. If anomalies are observed, further testing may be necessary, including sputum tests to identify the presence of the bacterium.

Interpreting Test Results: What They Mean

Understanding how to interpret TB test results is critical for patients and their families. A positive skin or blood test implies that the person has been exposed to TB bacteria; however, it does not determine whether the disease is active. For individuals who test positive, further assessment is necessary.

If chest X-rays suggest symptoms of active TB, or if sputum tests confirm the presence of Mycobacterium tuberculosis, the diagnosis of active TB is established. Conversely, persons with positive test results but normal X-rays may have latent TB, meaning they are infected but not contagious and do not develop symptoms.

Patients must engage together with healthcare providers to discuss their test results and understand the ramifications. An open communication can help ease anxiety and enable individuals to take control of their health journey.

Understanding Drug Resistance

One of the most serious issues in TB treatment is the rise of drug-resistant bacteria. Drug-resistant TB arises when the bacteria acquire resistance to the drugs generally used to treat the infection. This can happen for several causes, including insufficient treatment, incorrect medication, or a lack of adherence to the treatment plan.

Multidrug-Resistant TB (MDR-TB) is defined as TB that is resistant to at least isoniazid and rifampicin, the two most effective first-line TB treatments. Treating MDR-TB is more complex and involves a longer treatment duration, typically incorporating second-line drugs that can be less successful and more hazardous.

Extensively Drug-Resistant TB (XDR-TB) is an even more severe type, resistant to first-line treatments and many second-line choices. These situations are tough to handle and often require hospitalization and a complete, tailored treatment plan.

Understanding the implications of medication resistance is critical for patients. It emphasizes the necessity of adhering to prescribed treatments and having open communication with healthcare providers. Efforts to counteract medication resistance also include teaching on the need of finishing the complete course of therapy, even when symptoms improve.

The route to diagnosing tuberculosis is multidimensional, comprising a blend of clinical examination and multiple diagnostic modalities. Understanding the diagnostic process gives patients with the knowledge needed to interact meaningfully with their healthcare teams. As we shift to treatment alternatives, we will address how to properly manage TB and what support networks are crucial for navigating this challenging journey.

Overview of TB Medications and Regimens

Once identified, the path to recovery from tuberculosis entails a tough treatment regimen. The fundamental purpose of TB treatment is to remove the germs, restore health, and prevent the spread of the disease to others. The treatment procedure can seem daunting, but understanding the available options can empower patients and promote hope.

First-Line Medications:

The conventional treatment for drug-sensitive TB normally consists of a combination of first-line antibiotics administered over a six-month period. The core drugs include:

Isoniazid (INH): This antibiotic is particularly effective against TB bacteria and works by blocking cell wall formation.

Rifampicin (RIF): Rifampicin is another cornerstone of TB therapy, noted for its ability to destroy bacteria fast. It also prevents the establishment of drug resistance.

Ethambutol (EMB): Often used in the initial therapy phase, ethambutol helps prevent the development of resistance by targeting the bacteria's metabolism.

Pyrazinamide (PZA): This medication boosts the efficacy of the other treatments and is particularly useful in the initial phase of treatment.

The usual regimen consists of a two-month intensive phase with all four drugs, followed by a four-month continuation phase with isoniazid and rifampicin. Adherence to this schedule is crucial for effective treatment outcomes.

Second-Line Medications:

In cases of drug-resistant TB or when first-line treatments fail, second-line drugs are required. These can include fluoroquinolones, injectable medicines, and other antibiotics that are less often used. Treatment with second-line drugs can run for a year or longer, needing careful supervision to ensure the patient remains compliant and to monitor for side effects.

The Importance of Adherence to Treatment

Adhering to the approved TB treatment plan is vital for various reasons. First and foremost, it assures the effective elimination of the bacteria, lowering the danger of complications and long-term health difficulties. Additionally, constant adherence decreases the possibility of developing medication resistance, which complicates therapy and can have major public health concerns.

Challenges to Adherence:

Despite its importance, adherence to TB treatment can be tough. Side symptoms such as nausea, exhaustion, and probable liver damage can prevent patients from finishing their course. Additionally, the lengthy treatment duration might contribute to emotions of despondency, especially if symptoms improve before the course is completed.

To tackle these issues, healthcare providers can employ ways to support patients. Directly Observed Therapy (DOT) is one such strategy, where a healthcare provider supervises the patient as they take their medication. This strategy has proven helpful in improving adherence rates and assuring successful outcomes.

Managing Side Effects and Complications

Like any medical treatment, TB drugs come with potential adverse effects. Understanding this can help patients prepare and manage their experiences more successfully. Common side effects include:

Nausea and Gastrointestinal Discomfort: Many patients experience stomach upset, which can be controlled with dietary modifications or anti-nausea medicines.

Liver Toxicity: Some TB drugs, particularly isoniazid and rifampicin, might impact liver function. Regular monitoring through blood testing is vital to spot any concerns early.

Rash and Allergic responses: Skin responses may develop, and it is crucial for patients to report any odd symptoms to their healthcare professional.

Fatigue and Dizziness: These symptoms can occur, especially during the beginning periods of treatment. Patients should be advised to relax and stay hydrated.

For certain patients, problems may emerge, necessitating modifications to their treatment plan. Open communication with healthcare providers is crucial, allowing for rapid interventions and adjustments to improve tolerability.

The landscape of TB therapy is complex, requiring a detailed understanding of drugs, adherence techniques, and side effect management. By providing patients with knowledge, we may cultivate a sense of control over their treatment path. In the following chapter, we will review the key support networks accessible to those battling tuberculosis, highlighting the relevance of community, family, and healthcare services.

Role of Healthcare Providers

Navigating the road through tuberculosis treatment can be stressful, and the role of healthcare practitioners is important. From early diagnosis to recovery, these specialists serve as crucial guides, delivering medical expertise, emotional support, and practical counsel.

Healthcare practitioners, including doctors, nurses, and public health authorities, perform numerous vital roles:

Diagnosis and Treatment Planning: Providers are responsible for conducting tests, interpreting results, and devising tailored treatment plans based on each patient's needs.

Patient Education: Educating patients about TB, its transmission, and the importance of adherence to therapy is vital. Healthcare providers can demystify the disease, helping clients understand what to expect along their treatment path.

Monitoring Progress: Regular check-ups are important to assess therapy efficacy and handle any adverse effects or problems. Healthcare providers will do routine blood tests to check liver function and ensure that the drugs are working as planned.

Advocacy: Providers advocate for their patients, ensuring they have access to required resources and support services. This may involve referring patients to social assistance, mental health resources, or community programs.

Emotional and Psychological Support

Beyond the physical obstacles of TB, emotional and psychological support plays a key role in the recovery process. A diagnosis of tuberculosis can lead to feelings of fear, loneliness, and anxiety. It is crucial to address these emotional factors with the physical treatment to develop a comprehensive healing experience.

Counseling Services:

Many healthcare facilities offer counseling services to support individuals confronting chronic conditions. Licensed therapists can provide a safe space for patients to express their thoughts, address their anxieties, and create coping mechanisms. Cognitive-behavioral therapy (CBT) has been particularly beneficial in controlling anxiety and despair connected to chronic conditions.

Support Groups:

Help groups can also give vital emotional help. These events allow individuals to share their experiences, anxieties, and successes with others facing similar issues. The companionship and understanding that emerge among support groups can help individuals feel less alienated and more connected to others who understand their path.

Building a Support Network: Family, Friends, and Community Resources

In addition to healthcare doctors and mental health professionals, the support of family and friends is crucial for persons experiencing TB. Loved ones can offer practical aid, emotional encouragement, and a feeling of normalcy during a tough period.

Communicating Openly:

Encouraging open conversation about the disease can help family understand what their loved one is facing. This awareness can lead to increased empathy and support, creating a supportive atmosphere for healing.

Community Resources:

Many communities offer resources expressly geared at supporting individuals with tuberculosis. These may include transportation services for medical appointments, financial assistance programs for those confronting healthcare bills, and outreach initiatives that provide education and support to families affected by TB.

Organizations focused on public health and TB education can also be beneficial. They often give literature, workshops, and events geared at raising awareness about tuberculosis and connecting persons with the services they need.

Building a robust support system is crucial to the journey of combating tuberculosis. From healthcare providers to family and community supports, individuals do not have to confront this issue alone. As we continue to explore the nuances of TB, remember that assistance is accessible, and it is a critical aspect in navigating the complexity of diagnosis and treatment. Together, we will encourage hope and perseverance in the fight against tuberculosis.

Part III: Living with TB

Chapter 7: The Emotional Impact of TB

Coping with Diagnosis: Fear, Anxiety, and Stigma

Receiving a diagnosis of tuberculosis (TB) can be a life-altering experience, generally accompanied by a rush of emotions. The initial emotion is typically a blend of fear and worry. Fear of the unknown looms large: What will treatment involve? How will it influence my life? Will I be able to return to my normal routine? These inquiries can cause an overpowering sense of dread, leading individuals to address not just the disease itself but also the social ramifications related to it.

The stigma linked with TB can intensify these feelings. Even in today's linked world, myths regarding TB persist, leading to social ostracism and prejudice. People may be characterized as "infectious" or "unclean," aggravating the emotional load. This stigma might inhibit individuals from getting help, adhering to therapy, or sharing their experiences with others. The fear of judgment may lead to seclusion, worsening the psychological impact of the disease.

Strategies for Emotional Resilience

Coping with the emotional weight of a TB diagnosis demands a diverse strategy. Building emotional resilience is crucial to navigating this tough journey. Here are various ways that can help individuals regulate their feelings effectively:

Acknowledge Your Emotions:

It's crucial to acknowledge and validate the gamut of emotions you may be experiencing. Allow yourself to feel fear, grief, or anger without judgment. Acknowledgment is the first step toward processing these sentiments.

Seek Professional Help:

Engaging with a mental health professional can provide vital support. Therapists specialized in chronic illness management can give ways for managing with anxiety and sadness, helping clients create a positive mentality throughout their treatment path.

Connect with Others:

Building a support network is crucial. Share your feelings and experiences with trusted family members or friends who can offer understanding and encouragement. Support groups, both in-person and online, allow opportunity to interact with people facing similar issues. These relationships can help minimize feelings of loneliness and build a sense of community.

Practice Mindfulness and Relaxation Techniques:

Mindfulness techniques, such as meditation, deep breathing exercises, and yoga, can increase emotional well-being. These approaches help ground you in the current moment, minimizing concern about the future. Regular practice can build a sense of peace amidst the tumult.

Set Small Goals:

Focusing on tiny, achievable goals can instill a sense of purpose and success. Whether it's completing a chapter in a book or going for a brief stroll, appreciating these minor wins can enhance your happiness and maintain beneficial habits.

Educate Yourself:

Knowledge is power. Understanding TB, its treatment, and its ramifications helps ease anxiety associated with the unknown. The more informed you are, the more empowered you will feel in controlling your health.

Personal Stories of Hope and Recovery

To show the tenacity of individuals living with TB, we can draw inspiration from personal stories of hope and recovery.

Take the case of Maria, a young lady who faced a TB diagnosis at a key moment in her life. Initially overcome by terror, Maria felt lonely and condemned. However, after seeking help from a local TB organization, she connected with others who suffered similar experiences. This community empowered her to accept her journey. Maria put her dread into action, pushing for TB awareness in her community. Her tale shows the power of connection and the value of resilience in overcoming hardship.

Then there's Ahmed, a father of three, who was diagnosed with multidrug-resistant TB. Faced with an unknown future, Ahmed initially wrestled with sentiments of hopelessness. However, through treatment and assistance from his family, he learned to reinterpret his circumstances. Instead of perceiving his illness as a hindrance, he recognized it as a chance to improve his bond with his children. Ahmed shared his experiences freely with them, teaching them great lessons about health, resilience, and compassion.

These personal narratives serve as a reminder that even amid the darkest moments, hope and recovery are possible. By embracing their adventures, Maria and Ahmed not only found healing for themselves but also inspired others along the road.

Living with tuberculosis is obviously tough, but by addressing the emotional impact of the disease, individuals can grow resilience and foster hope. The stories of others who have confronted TB with fortitude remind us that we are not alone in our battles. In the following chapter, we will cover practical ways for navigating everyday life during treatment, ensuring that individuals can continue to live happy lives as they fight TB.

Managing Daily Routines During Treatment

Living with TB involves adaptations to regular habits, particularly during the treatment phase. While it may feel daunting, implementing tiny changes can lead to a more manageable and rewarding existence.

Establishing a Structured Routine:

Creating a regular regimen helps instill a sense of normalcy and control. Structure helps individuals keep focused on their health goals while ensuring that they don't neglect other crucial elements of life. Incorporate time for medication, meals, rest, and leisure activities.

Incorporating Treatment into Daily Life:

Adhering to a medicine schedule can be simpler by integrating it into existing routines. For instance, take prescriptions at the same time as meals or set reminders on your phone. Having a specific location for prescriptions can act as a visual reminder, underlining the significance of consistency.

Prioritizing Rest:

Fatigue can be a key challenge during TB therapy. Listen to your body and allow yourself appropriate rest. Short naps and relaxation practices help refresh both the mind and body, enabling better coping with treatment problems.

Balancing Responsibilities:

For individuals juggling job, family, and personal commitments, managing responsibilities can be intimidating. Communicate frankly with employers and family members about your needs. Many organizations offer flexible arrangements or accommodations for employees dealing with health concerns. Similarly, don't hesitate to call on family and friends for assistance with daily chores or childcare.

Nutrition and Lifestyle Changes for Recovery

Nutrition has a key part in healing from tuberculosis. A well-balanced diet bolsters the immune system, aids in healing, and helps lessen some negative effects of drugs. Here are crucial nutritional strategies:

Prioritize Nutrient-Dense Foods:

Incorporate a mix of fruits, vegetables, whole grains, and lean proteins into your diet. Foods rich in vitamins C and D, zinc, and antioxidants enhance immune function and overall health.

Stay Hydrated:

Maintaining sufficient hydration is vital, especially when using drugs that may lead to dehydration. Aim to drink plenty of water throughout the day. Herbal teas and clear broths can also be therapeutic.

Consult a Nutritionist:

For those struggling to navigate nutritional adjustments, consulting a nutritionist can provide individualized help. A nutritionist may assist build a food plan that matches with individual preferences and health needs, ensuring that necessary nutrients are addressed.

Staying Active and Maintaining Mental Health

Physical activity is an important component of rehabilitation from TB. While energy levels may fluctuate, finding methods to include movement into daily life will increase overall well-being. Here are some suggestions:

Gentle Exercise:

Engaging in low-impact activities such as walking, yoga, or stretching can increase physical strength and mental clarity. Even small spurts of action can raise mood and minimize feelings of weariness.

Mind-Body Practices:

Practices like yoga and tai chi integrate physical movement with mindfulness, fostering relaxation and emotional harmony. These exercises can help relieve stress, promote brain clarity, and improve overall happiness.

Prioritize Mental Health:

Maintaining mental health is as vital as physical health during TB treatment. Regularly engaging in things that provide joy—whether it's reading, crafts, or spending time in nature—can greatly increase emotional well-being.

Consider Therapy or Counseling:

For those facing serious anxiety or despair, therapy can give important help. A mental health expert can assist negotiate the emotional issues connected with TB, teaching techniques to promote resilience and manage with life's responsibilities.

Navigating everyday life while living with tuberculosis can be tough, but it is perfectly possible to maintain a full and balanced existence. By adopting disciplined routines, prioritizing nutrition, and finding ways to keep active, individuals can foster resilience and boost their overall well-being. In the last sections of this book, we will reflect on the journeys of those who have beaten TB, emphasizing optimism and the role of community in this struggle against the disease.

Part IV: Beyond Recovery

Chapter 9: Long-Term Health Considerations

Monitoring Health After Treatment

Completing treatment for tuberculosis (TB) is a tremendous milestone, although it signifies simply the beginning of a new journey toward long-term health and wellness. The shift from treatment to recovery involves sustained awareness and a proactive approach to health monitoring. Understanding how to navigate this new period is vital for preserving well-being and preventing difficulties.

Regular health check-ups are a crucial element of post-treatment care. Patients are asked to keep watchful about any lasting symptoms or new health issues that may occur. Symptoms such as chronic cough, unexplained weight loss, or weariness should be promptly reported with a healthcare physician, as they may suggest the need for further assessment. These continuing examinations serve a critical role in identifying potential issues early, allowing for appropriate intervention and management.

Possible Complications and Ongoing Care

While most persons recover well from TB, some may endure difficulties or residual effects. These problems might range from physical health issues to emotional and psychological challenges. Understanding these possibilities is crucial for everyone who has undergone TB treatment.

Respiratory Issues:

Some patients may continue to develop respiratory issues after completing TB treatment. This can emerge as a chronic cough, shortness of breath, or impaired lung function. Regular pulmonary function tests may be important to monitor lung health and detect any long-term repercussions of the condition.

Emotional and Psychological Health:

The emotional toll of a TB diagnosis and treatment can continue long after the physical symptoms have subsided. Anxiety, despair, or post-traumatic stress might be frequent, particularly for those who faced substantial health issues during treatment. Engaging with mental health specialists or support groups can provide vital coping methods and emotional support.

Preventive Health Measures:

Individuals who have had TB should focus preventive health practices. This involves taking vaccines (such as the flu shot), practicing excellent hygiene, and maintaining a healthy lifestyle through nutrition and exercise. A healthy lifestyle can increase immune function and lower the incidence of various infections.

The Importance of Follow-Up Appointments

Follow-up appointments are critical in the post-recovery phase, offering an opportunity for healthcare experts to examine the patient's overall health and treat any issues. These visits often involve extensive examinations, including physical exams, discussions of any persistent problems, and pulmonary function testing.

Patients should approach these appointments with a proactive mindset. Preparing questions in advance can assist guarantee that all issues are addressed. Additionally, maintaining a symptom diary can improve interactions with healthcare specialists, allowing for more accurate assessments.

In many circumstances, follow-up sessions will become less frequent over time, but patients should remain attentive and maintain an open channel of contact with their healthcare team. Regular contact with healthcare providers develops a sense of empowerment and encourages a proactive approach to long-term health.

Navigating the post-treatment phase of tuberculosis demands awareness and effort. By prioritizing health monitoring, understanding potential difficulties, and engaging in regular follow-up consultations, individuals can enhance their quality of life and lower the chance of future health challenges. In the following chapter, we will explore the power of advocacy and awareness in the fight against TB, concentrating on how individuals can make a difference for themselves and others in their communities.

How to Advocate for Yourself and Others

Advocacy plays a critical part in resolving the issues connected with tuberculosis, from boosting awareness to ensuring that persons receive the care they need. As a survivor or ally, you can become a significant voice in the fight against TB.

Understanding Your Rights:

Start by educating yourself on your rights as a patient. Familiarize yourself with healthcare policies, treatment options, and resources available to you. This knowledge helps you to advocate for yourself effectively and ensures that you receive the best possible care.

Effective Communication:

Being open and honest with healthcare providers is vital. Prepare for appointments by listing your symptoms, concerns, and questions. Clear communication can assist guarantee that your voice is heard and that you receive the required support and care.

Sharing Your Story:

Personal tales can be transformative in raising awareness and decreasing stigma. Sharing your story with TB—its struggles, victories, and lessons learned—can help others relate to your experience and inspire them to seek help. Whether through public speaking, social media, or community activities, your story can inspire others to confront TB with courage and perseverance.

The Role of Public Health Initiatives in TB Prevention

Public health programs have a key role in combating tuberculosis on a bigger scale. Understanding these activities and how you may participate will boost the success of the fight against TB.

Education and Awareness Campaigns:

Public health organizations routinely initiate education and awareness campaigns to enlighten populations about TB transmission, prevention, and treatment. These programs strive to eliminate myths and misconceptions while empowering individuals with knowledge. Engaging with these campaigns can build a sense of communal duty and collective action.

Screening and Prevention Programs:

Many health departments offer free or low-cost TB screenings, especially in high-risk communities. Participating in these initiatives can help identify instances early and reduce the spread of the disease. Encourage others to take use of these programs and promote screenings in your neighborhood.

Support for Advocacy Groups:

Consider getting active with local or national TB advocacy organizations. These groups generally provide information, education, and opportunities for community engagement. By joining forces with others who have a same objective, you may multiply your effect and contribute to significant change.

How to Get Involved in TB Awareness Campaigns

There are several ways to get involved in TB awareness initiatives, whether on a personal basis or through organized efforts. Here are some actionable measures you can take to make a difference:

Volunteer:

Offer your time to local health organizations, clinics, or TB advocacy groups. Volunteering can offer you with valuable insights and help you to interact with others who are concerned about TB awareness.

Social Media Advocacy:

Utilize social media tools to provide information about TB, advocate for awareness, and promote community health activities. Use hashtags, participate in campaigns, and share personal stories to reach a bigger audience.

Organize Events:

Consider arranging community events, such as health fairs, educational seminars, or awareness walks. Collaborating with local health professionals can boost the impact of these events and provide assistance to people in need.

Engage with Schools and Universities:

Partner with educational institutions to improve TB awareness among students. Educational workshops and seminars can develop a culture of awareness and empower future generations to take action.

Advocate for Policy Change:

Engage in advocacy efforts at the local or national level to affect healthcare policies related to TB prevention and treatment. This may involve calling out to lawmakers, engaging in advocacy days, or cooperating with existing advocacy organizations.

Advocacy and awareness are essential instruments in the fight against TB. By taking action—whether via personal advocacy, community participation, or public health initiatives—you can contribute to significant change and help establish a future where TB is no longer a concern. In the last chapter, we will look forward to the future of TB research and treatment, analyzing emerging trends and breakthroughs that offer the promise of a healthy tomorrow.

The Future of TB Research and Treatment

As we stand on the brink of substantial achievements in the fight against tuberculosis, the future appears optimistic. Ongoing research is crucial to creating more effective treatments, vaccines, and methods for treating TB on a worldwide basis.

Innovative Treatment Approaches:

Recent breakthroughs in TB research have led to the testing of innovative treatment regimens, including shorter and more effective antibiotic treatments. These developments can enhance treatment adherence and lower the likelihood of medication resistance, ultimately leading to better patient outcomes.

Vaccine Development:

The quest for a more effective TB vaccination has gathered steam in recent years. Several candidates are now in clinical studies, seeking to boost protection against TB. A effective vaccine might change TB prevention and substantially lower infection rates worldwide.

Personalized Medicine:

The future of TB treatment may possibly incorporate personalized medicine approaches, modifying medicines based on specific patient needs and genetic characteristics. This focused technique can lead to more effective and efficient treatment programs, decreasing side effects and boosting overall success rates.

Emerging Trends and Innovations in TB Care

The landscape of TB care is always shifting, with growing trends and ideas that promise to transform how we handle the disease.

Telemedicine and Remote Monitoring:

The rise of telemedicine has changed healthcare delivery, particularly in underprivileged areas. Remote consultations and monitoring can increase access to care, allowing patients to contact with healthcare experts from the comfort of their homes. This tendency is particularly advantageous for persons suffering issues linked to transportation or mobility.

Community-Based Approaches:

Recognizing the importance of community in healthcare, several organizations are embracing community-based methods to TB prevention and treatment. Engaging community health workers to provide information, screenings, and support develops trust and encourages folks to seek care.

Technology and Data Analytics:

Advancements in technology and data analytics are playing a vital role in understanding and fighting TB. Using data to track infection trends, identify high-risk populations, and adapt interventions can boost the success of public health activities.

Empowering Future Generations Against TB

Empowering future generations to tackle tuberculosis is vital for guaranteeing a healthier tomorrow. Education and awareness are essential components in building resilience against TB and promoting a culture of health.

Educational Initiatives:

Integrating TB teaching into school curricula can create awareness from an early age. Teaching children about TB transmission, prevention, and treatment can help demystify the disease and eliminate stigma, producing a more informed and empathctic society.

Engaging Youth in Advocacy:

Encouraging young people to get part in advocacy and awareness initiatives can amplify their voices in the fight against TB. Providing chances for adolescents to participate in community activities, research projects, and public speaking engagements can empower them to be agents of change.

Inspiring a Global Movement:

As we look to the future, the fight against TB demands a collective effort that spans borders. Inspiring a worldwide movement focused on prevention, treatment, and research may unite individuals, organizations, and governments in the shared goal of eradicating TB.

The future of tuberculosis care is loaded with optimism and possibility. By embracing innovative research, increasing community participation, and empowering future generations, we can pave the road for a world where TB no longer poses a danger. Together, we can fight this sickness with insight and optimism, building a healthy future for everybody. As we complete this trip through the challenges and successes of tuberculosis, remember that each step made in awareness, campaigning, and research takes us closer to a world free from TB.

Conclusion

As we draw to a close on this voyage through the diverse environment of tuberculosis (TB), it is necessary to reflect on the major messages that reverberate throughout the pages of this book: hope, resilience, and the power of knowledge. These themes serve not only as cornerstones in the fight against TB but also as guiding concepts for personal growth and communal health.

Hope: A Light in the Darkness

The story of TB is typically entwined with fear and stigma, originating from a lack of awareness about the disease and its impact on individuals and communities. However, as we have explored, optimism shines brilliantly even in the most stressful circumstances.   The stories of tenacity, recovery, and triumph over hardship remind us that healing is possible.

Hope is not only a passive sentiment; it is an active energy that moves individuals and society forward. It is the belief that, despite the hurdles we confront, a better tomorrow is achievable. The improvements in TB research, treatment choices, and community engagement efforts give a good foundation for this hope. Each step forward in understanding and combating TB underscores the belief that we are capable of change, both individually and collectively.

Consider the folks who have bravely shared their stories throughout this book. Their adventures are tribute to the resilience of the human spirit in conquering the hurdles offered by TB. Each personal account exemplifies the idea that hope may thrive in the face of hardship. It is this hope that feeds activism, inspires action, and pushes others to seek aid and support.

Resilience: The Strength Within

Resilience is another significant element that underlies our understanding of TB. Resilience is not merely the ability to resist adversities; it is the capability to grow and adapt in response to adversity. The journey through TB—whether as a patient, caregiver, or community advocate—requires great resilience.

Throughout the chapters, we have dug into the emotional and psychological implications of a

TB diagnosis, noting the fear and anxiety that typically accompany such news. However, we have also highlighted ways for strengthening emotional resilience, emphasizing the need of self-care, support networks, and coping mechanisms. The ability to bounce back from setbacks, to find strength in weakness, and to seek help when needed are essential components of resilience.

As we embrace resilience, it is crucial to remember that we are not alone in our problems. Communities are strong sources of support, and by developing connections and sharing experiences, we may uplift one another. Engaging with support groups, participating in community activities, and sharing personal stories create a network of strength that empowers us all.

The Power of Knowledge

Knowledge is a vital instrument in the struggle against TB. Throughout this book, we have stressed the necessity of understanding TB—its transmission, symptoms, diagnosis, treatment options, and the ongoing need for vigilance in health monitoring. Empowering individuals with knowledge supports informed decision-making, minimizes stigma, and encourages proactive health habits.

As we traverse the complexity of TB, it is vital to be informed on the newest research, treatment developments, and public health measures.

Knowledge not only helps individuals speak for themselves but also allows communities to challenge disinformation and create awareness. By sharing knowledge and educating others, we contribute to a culture of understanding and empathy that helps break down barriers and eliminate the stigma associated with TB.

Taking Action for Personal and Community Health

As we complete this book, I encourage everyone of you to take action—whether for your personal health or the health of your community. Action starts with awareness and education. Here are few practical things you may take to make a difference:

Educate Yourself and Others:

Stay informed on TB, its symptoms, and preventative strategies. Share this knowledge with friends, family, and your community. Consider conducting educational workshops or talks to stimulate dialogue about TB and refute myths.

Advocate for Health:

Become an advocate for TB awareness and treatment access in your town. Engage with local health organizations, participate in awareness campaigns, and support efforts that encourage TB tests and education.

Support Those Affected by TB:

If you know someone who has been afflicted by TB, show your support. Whether via emotional encouragement, practical assistance, or simply being a listening ear, your presence can make a huge impact in their path.

Prioritize Your Health:

If you have a history of TB or any respiratory difficulties, emphasize frequent health check-ups and screenings. Staying diligent about your health and obtaining medical assistance when needed is vital for long-term well-being.

Engage with Community Resources:

Explore local resources for TB education and assistance. Many health authorities and organizations offer free or low-cost screenings, information sessions, and support groups. Participating in these resources can strengthen your understanding and connection to your community.

Empower Future Generations:

Work to guarantee that future generations are knowledgeable about TB and empowered to take action. Engage with schools, youth organizations, and community centers to promote education and awareness among young people.

Promote Research and Innovation:

Advocate for continuing funding and support for TB research and innovation. The breakthroughs in treatment and preventative techniques rely on continuing research initiatives that require public support and engagement.

Foster a Culture of Compassion:

Combat stigma by building a culture of compassion and understanding in your community. Challenge myths and encourage open discussions about TB.

A Call to Action

The struggle against tuberculosis is far from ended, but the progress we have made thus far is a monument to the power of hope, resilience, and knowledge. Each of us has a role to play in this journey, whether as individuals, caregivers, activists, or community members. By embracing these principles and taking action, we can contribute to a healthy world—one where TB no longer holds the ability to instill dread and uncertainty.

In closing, realize that you are not alone. The stories of hope and perseverance we have examined throughout this book reflect the voices of countless others who have endured TB. Together, we can continue to break down barriers, promote awareness, and support one another in this essential goal.

Let us move forward with courage and conviction, armed with information and a shared commitment to health and well-being. The path may be tough, but it is also packed with the promise of a brighter future—a future where we confront TB not with fear, but with hope and determination. Thank you for joining me on this journey, and may we all strive together to establish a world free from the burdens of tuberculosis.

The end